EAT

FOR

YOUR AGE

The Complete Guide to Nutrition Throughout Your Life

2nd Edition

By

Dr. Michael McCoy

i

Contents

INTRODUCTION
WHY YOUR AGE MATTERS MORE THAN YOU THINK

Let me start with a story that changed how I think about nutrition forever.

Two years ago, I met Margaret, a vibrant 72-year-old who looked and acted twenty years younger than her age. She had energy that put my younger patients to shame, a sharp mind, and the kind of glowing health that made people stop and ask, "What's your secret?"

The same week, I met David, a 45-year-old executive who looked exhausted, struggled with his weight, and was already on medications for high blood pressure and diabetes. He was frustrated because despite following the same "healthy eating" advice everyone gets, he felt worse every year.

What was the difference? Margaret had learned something that David hadn't: your nutritional needs change dramatically as you age, and what works at 25 can actually work against you at 45, 65, or 85.

After thirty years as a doctor specializing in nutrition and preventive medicine, I've seen this pattern repeatedly. The people who age successfully—who stay energetic, healthy, and independent well into their 80s and 90s—aren't necessarily the ones who follow generic healthy eating advice. They're the ones who understand that eating for your age is just as important as eating for your health.

This book will show you exactly what that means for your life right now, and how to adjust your eating as you move through each decade. No complicated meal plans or impossible-to-follow diets. Just practical, science-based guidance that acknowledges a simple truth: your 25-year-old body has different needs than your 45-year-old body, which has different needs than your 65-year-old body.

Let's start this journey together.

CHAPTER 1
THE SCIENCE BEHIND EATING FOR YOUR AGE (MADE SIMPLE)

Why One Size Doesn't Fit All Ages

Think about your car for a moment. You wouldn't use the same maintenance routine for a brand-new car that you'd use for a 15-year-old vehicle, right? The newer car might need premium gas and regular oil changes, while the older one might need special additives, more frequent tune-ups, and different types of care to keep running smoothly.

Your body works the same way. A 25-year-old body is like that new car—it can handle almost anything you throw at it and bounce back quickly. But a 55-year-old body is more like a well-maintained older car that needs more specific care to perform its best.

Here's what happens inside your body as you age, explained in terms anyone can understand:

Your Body's Internal Changes Over Time

Your Digestive System Becomes Pickier

Remember being able to eat pizza at midnight in college without any problems? That's because young digestive systems produce plenty of stomach acid and digestive enzymes. But as we age, our stomach produces less acid—about 25% less by age 60. This means we don't absorb nutrients from food as easily, especially important ones like vitamin B12, iron, and calcium.

Recent research from Harvard's School of Public Health found that this change starts as early as our 30s, which explains why so many people start having digestive issues in their 40s and 50s that they never had before.

Your Metabolism Hits the Brakes

Your metabolism—the rate at which your body burns calories—naturally slows down as you age. But here's what's interesting: it's not just about getting older. It's mostly about losing muscle mass. Every decade after 30, you lose about 3-8% of your muscle mass if you don't actively work to prevent it.

Muscle tissue burns calories even when you're sitting still, so less muscle means fewer calories burned throughout the day. This is why people often gain weight in their 40s and 50s even when they're eating the same amount they always have.

Your Hormones Start Playing by Different Rules

Hormones are like your body's internal messaging system, and as we age, some of these messages change. Growth hormone levels drop, making it harder to build and maintain muscle. Insulin becomes less effective, making it harder to control blood sugar. For women, estrogen levels plummet during menopause, affecting everything from bone health to where fat gets stored.

These changes aren't inevitable decline—they're signals that your body needs different support to function optimally.

The Good News: You Have More Control Than You Think

Here's what excites me most about the research coming out of major universities and medical centers around the world: the right nutrition can dramatically slow down, stop, or even reverse many age-related changes.

Scientists at Yale University recently completed a study that followed 1,200 people over 20 years. They found that people who adjusted their eating habits to match their changing nutritional needs maintained their physical and mental function much better than those who didn't. The difference was so significant that at age 75, the people who "ate for their age" had the physical capabilities of typical 60-year-olds.

The Three Key Principles of Age-Appropriate Nutrition

Based on decades of research and my experience with thousands of patients, eating for your age comes down to three fundamental principles:

1. Nutrient Density Becomes More Important

When you're young, you can afford to "waste" some calories on foods that don't provide much nutrition. But as your calorie needs decrease with age, every bite needs to count more. This doesn't mean eating less—it means eating smarter.

2. Protein Requirements Actually Increase

Contrary to popular belief, older adults need more protein, not less. While a 25-year-old might thrive on 50-60 grams of protein per day, a 65-year-old needs 75-100 grams to maintain muscle mass and strength.

3. Timing Matters More

Young bodies are forgiving about when you eat. Older bodies perform better with more consistent meal timing and specific nutrient timing around physical activity.

What This Means for You

Throughout this book, I'll show you exactly how to apply these principles to your current age and situation. You don't need to become a nutrition expert or completely overhaul your life. Small, targeted changes based on your age can produce dramatic improvements in how you feel and function.

The goal isn't to stop aging—it's to age successfully. And that journey starts with understanding that your nutritional needs aren't the same at 45 as they were at 25, and they won't be the same at 65 as they are today.

CHAPTER 2
YOUR BODY'S CHANGING NEEDS: WHAT HAPPENS AS WE AGE

The Decade-by-Decade Breakdown

Let me walk you through what happens in your body during each decade of life, and why these changes matter for how you should eat.

Your 20s and 30s: The Building Phase

What's Happening in Your Body:

This is your biological prime time. Your body is like a construction site in the best possible way—building bone density, muscle mass, and establishing the cellular foundations that will carry you through the rest of your life.

Dr. Sarah Johnson at Stanford University's Longevity Center calls this the "biological investment period." The nutritional choices you make now are like making deposits in a health savings account that you'll draw from for the next 50+ years.

Key Changes:

- **Bone Building**: 90% of your lifetime bone mass is built by age 30
- **Peak Muscle**: You reach maximum muscle mass and strength

- **Hormonal Prime**: Growth hormone, testosterone, and estrogen are at optimal levels
- **Fast Recovery**: Your body repairs itself quickly from stress, poor sleep, or dietary mistakes

The Hidden Challenge: This efficiency can work against you. Because your body is so good at compensating for poor choices, it's easy to develop habits that will cause problems later. Think of it as your body writing checks that your future self will have to cash.

Your 40s: The Transition Phase

What's Happening in Your Body:

This is when your body starts sending you subtle messages that things are changing. You might notice that you can't eat the same foods you used to without gaining weight, or that you need more sleep to feel rested, or that stress affects you differently.

Research from the Mayo Clinic shows that this decade is crucial because it's when many chronic diseases begin developing, even if you don't have symptoms yet.

Key Changes:

- **Metabolism Slowdown**: Your calorie-burning rate decreases by about 5% per decade
- **Hormone Shifts**: Growth hormone and sex hormones begin declining
- **Muscle Loss Begins**: You start losing 3-8% of muscle mass per decade

- **Insulin Resistance**: Your cells become less responsive to insulin
- **Increased Inflammation**: Your body's background inflammation levels rise

The Opportunity: This is the perfect time to make changes because your body still responds quickly to improvements in diet and lifestyle.

Your 50s and 60s: The Prevention Phase

What's Happening in Your Body:

This is when the changes become more noticeable, but it's also when targeted nutrition can have its biggest impact. Many of my patients tell me they feel better in their 60s than they did in their 40s once they learn how to eat for their age.

A landmark study from Harvard followed 78,000 women for 14 years and found that those who made specific dietary adjustments in their 50s had a 40% lower risk of chronic disease in their 70s compared to those who didn't.

Key Changes:

- **Menopause/Andropause**: Major hormonal shifts affect metabolism, bone health, and body composition
- **Absorption Issues**: Decreased stomach acid makes it harder to absorb certain nutrients
- **Increased Disease Risk**: Higher likelihood of diabetes, heart disease, and osteoporosis

- **Slower Recovery**: It takes longer to bounce back from illness or stress
- **Cognitive Changes**: Some decline in processing speed and memory

The Power Period: Despite these challenges, this is when proper nutrition can be most transformative. Your body is still capable of remarkable improvements with the right support.

Your 70s and Beyond: The Maintenance Phase

What's Happening in Your Body:

This phase is about maintaining independence, strength, and cognitive function. The good news is that people who eat appropriately for this life stage often surprise their doctors—and themselves—with their vitality.

Dr. Robert Butler, who pioneered the field of aging research, found that proper nutrition could help people maintain the physical function of someone 10-15 years younger.

Key Changes:

- **Appetite Reduction**: Natural decrease in hunger signals
- **Taste and Smell Changes**: Foods may seem less flavorful
- **Medication Interactions**: Multiple prescriptions can affect nutrient absorption
- **Social Eating Challenges**: Cooking for one, limited mobility, or isolation

- **Increased Protein Needs**: Despite smaller appetites, protein requirements actually increase

The Wisdom Advantage: While there are challenges, this is also when people often have more time and motivation to focus on their health, leading to remarkable improvements.

The Common Thread: Adaptation is Key

What I've learned from treating patients of all ages is that the people who age most successfully are those who adapt their eating to match their body's changing needs. They don't try to eat like they're 25 when they're 55, and they don't resign themselves to decline when they're 75.

Individual Variation: Why Your Mileage May Vary

While these general patterns hold true for most people, everyone ages differently. Genetics, lifestyle, stress levels, and medical history all play a role. Some 70-year-olds have the nutritional needs of typical 50-year-olds, while some 50-year-olds need strategies usually recommended for older adults.

The key is paying attention to how your body responds to different foods and eating patterns, and adjusting accordingly. In the coming chapters, I'll give you specific guidance for each age range, along with signs that you might need to modify the recommendations for your individual situation.

CHAPTER 3
THE POWER OF FOOD AS MEDICINE

How Food Fights Aging from the Inside Out

Before we dive into specific recommendations for each age group, I want to share something that might change how you think about food forever: every bite you take is either fighting aging or accelerating it. There's really no neutral ground.

This isn't just philosophical—it's measurable. Scientists can now look at your cells and determine your biological age versus your chronological age. Some 60-year-olds have the cellular age of 45-year-olds, while some 45-year-olds have the cellular age of 60-year-olds. The difference often comes down to lifestyle choices, with nutrition being the biggest factor.

The Anti-Aging Nutrients Your Body Craves

Antioxidants: Your Cellular Bodyguards

Think of antioxidants as your body's cleanup crew. Every day, your cells produce waste products called free radicals—it's a normal part of being alive, like how a car produces exhaust. But as we age, we produce more of these free radicals and our natural cleanup systems become less efficient.

Free radicals damage your cells, contributing to everything from wrinkles to heart disease to memory problems. Antioxidants neutralize these free radicals before they can cause damage.

The exciting research happening at universities like Johns Hopkins and UCLA shows that people who eat antioxidant-rich foods consistently have measurably younger-looking cells and better function across all body systems.

The Best Food Sources:

- **Berries**: Blueberries, strawberries, and blackberries top the charts
- **Dark leafy greens**: Spinach, kale, and Swiss chard
- **Colorful vegetables**: The deeper the color, the more antioxidants
- **Green tea**: Contains powerful compounds called catechins
- **Dark chocolate**: 70% cacao or higher provides flavonoids

Omega-3 Fatty Acids: Your Brain's Best Friend

If antioxidants are your cellular bodyguards, omega-3 fatty acids are your brain's maintenance crew. These essential fats keep your brain cells flexible and healthy, reduce inflammation throughout your body, and support heart health.

Dr. Martha Clare Morris at Rush University conducted a study of 900 people over six years and found that those who ate fish rich in omega-3s at least once a week had significantly slower cognitive decline. The difference was equivalent to being 3-4 years younger mentally.

The Best Sources:

- **Fatty fish**: Salmon, sardines, mackerel, and anchovies

- **Walnuts**: One of the best plant sources
- **Flaxseeds**: Grind them fresh for maximum benefit
- **Chia seeds**: Easy to add to smoothies or yogurt

Protein: Your Muscle's Foundation

Here's something that surprises many people: as you age, you actually need more protein, not less. Young adults can maintain their muscle mass on about 0.8 grams of protein per kilogram of body weight. But adults over 50 need 1.2-1.6 grams per kilogram to prevent muscle loss.

Why does this matter? Muscle isn't just about looking strong—it's about staying independent. Muscle mass is directly linked to your ability to climb stairs, carry groceries, recover from illness, and maintain your balance to prevent falls.

Quality Matters:

- **Complete proteins**: Contain all essential amino acids your body can't make
- **Easily digestible**: Especially important as stomach acid decreases with age
- **Well-distributed**: Spread protein throughout the day rather than loading up at one meal

The Inflammation Connection

One of the biggest discoveries in aging research over the past decade is the role of chronic inflammation. Unlike the inflammation you get from an injury (which is helpful for healing), chronic inflammation is like having a small fire burning inside your body all the time.

This low-level inflammation contributes to heart disease, diabetes, arthritis, Alzheimer's disease, and even depression. The good news is that certain foods can dramatically reduce this inflammation, while others can increase it.

Anti-Inflammatory Superstars:

- **Fatty fish**: The omega-3s directly reduce inflammatory markers
- **Olive oil**: Contains compounds that work like natural anti-inflammatory drugs
- **Turmeric**: The compound curcumin is incredibly powerful against inflammation
- **Tart cherries**: Natural compounds that reduce inflammation and improve sleep
- **Leafy greens**: Packed with inflammation-fighting nutrients

Inflammation Promoters to Limit:

- **Processed foods**: High in chemicals that trigger inflammation
- **Sugar**: Spikes blood sugar and promotes inflammatory responses
- **Trans fats**: Found in some margarines and processed foods
- **Excessive alcohol**: More than moderate amounts increase inflammation

- **Refined carbohydrates**: White bread, pastries, and sugary snacks

Intermittent Fasting: The Reset Button for Your Cells

One of the most exciting developments in anti-aging nutrition is research on intermittent fasting. This isn't about starving yourself—it's about giving your digestive system regular breaks so your body can focus on cellular cleanup and repair.

Dr. Valter Longo at USC has published groundbreaking research showing that periodic fasting triggers a process called autophagy, where your cells essentially "take out the trash" by recycling damaged components and clearing out toxins.

Simple Approaches:

- **16:8 Method**: Eat within an 8-hour window, fast for 16 hours (including sleep)
- **5:2 Approach**: Eat normally 5 days, reduce calories to 500-600 on 2 days
- **Overnight fasting**: Simply extend the time between dinner and breakfast

Important Note: Fasting isn't appropriate for everyone. People with diabetes, eating disorders, or certain medical conditions should consult their doctor first.

Hydration: The Most Overlooked Anti-Aging Tool

As we age, our sense of thirst becomes less reliable, and our kidneys become less efficient at conserving water. Yet proper hydration affects everything from skin appearance to brain function to joint health.

Researchers at Loma Linda University found that people who drank adequate water had significantly better cognitive function and were less likely to develop heart disease compared to those who were chronically mildly dehydrated.

How Much is Enough:

- **General rule**: Half your body weight in ounces (150 pounds = 75 ounces)
- **Quality counts**: Clean, filtered water is best
- **Timing matters**: Sip throughout the day rather than chugging large amounts
- **Food sources**: Fruits and vegetables provide about 20% of fluid needs

Making Food Your Medicine Cabinet

The beauty of eating for your age is that food becomes your first line of defense against aging. Instead of waiting for problems to develop and then treating them with medications, you're actively preventing issues while nourishing your body optimally.

This doesn't mean you'll never need medical care—genetics and other factors play important roles in health. But it does mean you're stacking the deck in your favor and giving yourself the best possible chance to age successfully.

In the next chapters, I'll show you exactly how to put these principles into practice for your specific age and situation.

CHAPTER 4
THE BUILDING YEARS (20S TO 30S) - SETTING YOURSELF UP FOR LIFE

The Investment Decade

If I could sit down with every person in their 20s and 30s, here's what I'd tell them: this is your investment decade. The nutritional choices you make now will determine how you feel and function for the next 50+ years. It's like compound interest for your health.

I know that might sound dramatic when you feel invincible and can bounce back from almost anything, but bear with me. The patients I see who are thriving in their 70s and 80s almost universally made good nutritional choices in their younger years, while those struggling with multiple health issues often trace their problems back to habits established in their 20s and 30s.

Your Body's Biological To-Do List

During these decades, your body is working on several major projects:

Building Your Peak Bone Mass

Think of your bones like a savings account. You can only make deposits until about age 30, after which you can only maintain or withdraw. By age 30, you'll have accumulated about 90% of your lifetime bone mass. This foundation will determine whether you have strong bones in your 70s or face fractures and osteoporosis.

Research from the National Institutes of Health shows that people who optimize their bone-building nutrition in their 20s have 40% lower fracture risk in their later years.

Establishing Your Metabolic Baseline

Your metabolism during these years sets the pattern for the rest of your life. People who maintain stable blood sugar and healthy body composition in their 20s and 30s have much easier time avoiding diabetes and weight gain as they age.

Creating Your Muscle Mass Peak

You'll reach your maximum muscle mass sometime in your 30s. While you can build muscle at any age, it's much easier to maintain what you have than to rebuild what you've lost.

The Unique Challenges of This Age Group

The Busy Life Problem

Most people in their 20s and 30s are juggling demanding careers, relationships, possibly young children, and social lives. Healthy eating often takes a backseat to convenience, leading to patterns that become harder to break over time.

The Invincibility Trap

Your body is incredibly forgiving during these years. You can skip meals, eat junk food, drink too much, and get too little sleep without immediate consequences. This can create a false sense that these choices don't matter—but they're accumulating interest that you'll pay later.

The Information Overload

This is the age when people are most likely to try extreme diets, follow contradictory advice from social media, and get caught up in nutrition trends that may not be based on solid science.

Your Nutritional Priorities for Maximum Impact

Priority #1: Build Unshakeable Bones

What you need:

- **Calcium**: 1,000mg daily (about 3 servings of dairy or calcium-rich foods)
- **Vitamin D**: 800-1,000 IU daily (from sun exposure, food, or supplements)
- **Vitamin K2**: 100-200mcg daily (from fermented foods or supplements)
- **Magnesium**: 400mg daily for men, 310mg for women
- **Protein**: 1.2-1.6g per kg of body weight to support bone matrix

Best food sources:

- **Dairy products**: Milk, yogurt, cheese (choose low-fat varieties)
- **Leafy greens**: Kale, collard greens, bok choy

- **Sardines and canned salmon with bones**: Excellent calcium and vitamin D
- **Almonds and sesame seeds**: Good plant sources of calcium
- **Fortified plant milks**: If you don't consume dairy

Real-world tip: If you're not a big milk drinker, try adding Greek yogurt to smoothies, using cheese in salads, or drinking calcium-fortified plant milk.

Priority #2: Optimize Your Reproductive Health

Whether you're planning to have children now or in the future, these nutrients are crucial:

For Women:

- **Folate**: 400-800mcg daily to prevent birth defects
- **Iron**: 18mg daily to replace losses from menstruation
- **Omega-3s**: 200-300mg DHA daily for brain development

For Men:

- **Zinc**: 11mg daily for healthy sperm production
- **Antioxidants**: Vitamin C, E, and selenium to protect sperm quality
- **Folate**: Yes, men need it too for healthy sperm

Best sources:

- **Folate**: Dark leafy greens, beans, fortified cereals, oranges
- **Iron**: Lean red meat, poultry, fish, beans, spinach

- **Zinc**: Oysters, lean meat, pumpkin seeds, chickpeas

Priority #3: Establish Stable Blood Sugar Patterns

The eating patterns you establish now will determine your diabetes risk for life. People who maintain stable blood sugar in their 20s and 30s are much less likely to develop type 2 diabetes later.

Key strategies:

- **Eat protein at every meal**: Helps stabilize blood sugar
- **Choose complex carbohydrates**: Whole grains, beans, vegetables
- **Don't skip meals**: Irregular eating patterns promote insulin resistance
- **Watch portion sizes**: Even healthy foods can spike blood sugar in large amounts

Sample daily eating pattern:

- **Breakfast**: Greek yogurt with berries and nuts
- **Lunch**: Salad with grilled chicken, quinoa, and olive oil dressing
- **Snack**: Apple with almond butter
- **Dinner**: Baked fish, roasted vegetables, brown rice

Special Considerations for Your 20s and 30s

If You're Very Active:

Athletes and very active people have higher needs for:

- **Protein**: 1.6-2.2g per kg body weight
- **Carbohydrates**: 5-7g per kg body weight on training days
- **Iron**: Especially important for endurance athletes
- **B vitamins**: Higher needs due to increased energy metabolism

If You're Vegetarian or Vegan:

Pay special attention to:

- **Vitamin B12**: 2.4mcg daily (must supplement)
- **Iron**: Eat with vitamin C to improve absorption
- **Zinc**: Found in beans, nuts, seeds, whole grains
- **Omega-3s**: From algae supplements if not eating fish
- **Complete proteins**: Combine rice and beans, or use quinoa

If You Drink Alcohol Regularly:

Alcohol interferes with nutrient absorption and increases needs for:

- **B vitamins**: Especially thiamine, folate, and B12
- **Magnesium**: Alcohol increases losses
- **Antioxidants**: To combat alcohol-related oxidative stress

Practical limits: No more than 1 drink daily for women, 2 for men, with at least 2 alcohol-free days per week.

Simple Daily Habits That Pay Huge Dividends

The 5-a-Day Foundation

Aim for at least 5 servings of fruits and vegetables daily, but think variety over quantity. Different colors provide different protective compounds.

Monday: Red (tomatoes, red peppers, strawberries) **Tuesday**: Orange (carrots, sweet potatoes, oranges) **Wednesday**: Yellow (squash, corn, bananas) **Thursday**: Green (broccoli, spinach, kiwi) **Friday**: Blue/Purple (blueberries, eggplant, purple cabbage)

The Protein-at-Every-Meal Rule

Include 20-30g of protein at each meal to maintain muscle mass and stable blood sugar:

- **Breakfast**: 2 eggs or 1 cup Greek yogurt
- **Lunch**: 4 oz chicken breast or 1 cup beans
- **Dinner**: 4-6 oz fish or tofu

The Healthy Fat Focus

Include healthy fats at every meal to support hormone production and nutrient absorption:

- **Avocado**: 1/4 to 1/2 per day
- **Nuts and seeds**: 1 oz (small handful) daily
- **Olive oil**: 1-2 tablespoons for cooking or salads
- **Fatty fish**: 2-3 servings per week

Warning Signs You Need to Adjust Your Approach

Energy Issues:

- Constant fatigue despite adequate sleep
- Need for caffeine to function
- Energy crashes in the afternoon

Digestive Problems:

- Frequent bloating or gas
- Irregular bowel movements
- Heartburn or acid reflux

Mood and Sleep Changes:

- Difficulty falling or staying asleep
- Mood swings or irritability
- Difficulty concentrating

Physical Changes:

- Unexplained weight gain or loss
- Frequent colds or infections
- Slow healing from cuts or injuries

If you're experiencing any of these consistently, it may be time to work with a healthcare provider to evaluate your nutritional status and make adjustments.

The Bottom Line for Your 20s and 30s

This is your time to build the strongest possible foundation for the decades ahead. You don't need to be perfect, but you do need to be consistent. Small, sustainable changes made now will compound over time into dramatically better health as you age.

Focus on the big picture: eat mostly whole foods, include protein at every meal, get plenty of fruits and vegetables, stay hydrated, and don't let perfect be the enemy of good. Your future self will thank you.

CHAPTER 5
THE SHIFTING YEARS (40S) - WHEN YOUR BODY STARTS CHANGING

The Wake-Up Call Decade

Welcome to your 40s—the decade when your body starts sending you gentle (and sometimes not-so-gentle) reminders that you're not 25 anymore. This is when many of my patients first come to see me, frustrated because the eating and exercise habits that used to work just fine are suddenly letting them down.

"I haven't changed anything about how I eat," they tell me, "but I'm gaining weight and feeling tired all the time."

Here's what I tell them: you haven't changed, but your body has. And that's completely normal. The good news is that once you understand these changes and adjust your approach accordingly, many people feel better in their late 40s than they did in their early 40s.

What's Really Happening in Your 40s

Your Metabolism Officially Hits the Brakes

Remember how you could eat pizza at midnight in your 20s without consequence? Those days are officially over. Your metabolism slows by about 5% per decade, and this is the decade when most people really start to notice it.

But here's what's interesting: it's not just about burning fewer calories. Your body also starts preferentially storing fat around your midsection instead of your hips and thighs. This happens because of hormonal changes, particularly a gradual decline in growth hormone and changes in insulin sensitivity.

Your Hormones Start Playing by Different Rules

This is when the hormonal symphony that's been playing smoothly for decades starts to hit some off notes:

- **Growth hormone**: Begins declining, making it harder to build and maintain muscle
- **Insulin sensitivity**: Decreases, making it easier to store fat and harder to control blood sugar
- **Sex hormones**: Begin fluctuating (women) or gradually declining (men)
- **Cortisol**: Often becomes elevated due to increased life stress
- **Thyroid function**: May begin to slow down

Your Body's Repair Systems Slow Down

Your body's ability to repair damage from stress, poor sleep, or dietary indiscretions becomes less efficient. This is why a night of drinking affects you more than it used to, why you need more sleep to feel rested, and why minor injuries take longer to heal.

The Hidden Opportunities of Your 40s

While these changes might sound discouraging, your 40s actually present unique opportunities for health improvement:

Your Brain is Hitting Its Peak

Research from MIT shows that many cognitive abilities peak in your 40s, including the ability to understand complex information and make good decisions. This makes it an ideal time to master nutrition principles that will serve you for life.

You Have More Control Over Your Environment

Unlike your 20s and 30s, when you might have been at the mercy of cafeteria food, tight budgets, or chaotic schedules, most people in their 40s have more control over what they eat and when they eat it.

Small Changes Have Big Impact

Your body becomes more responsive to targeted interventions. The right dietary changes can produce noticeable improvements in energy, weight, and overall health within weeks.

Your New Nutritional Priorities

Priority #1: Reboot Your Metabolism

The key to maintaining a healthy weight and energy level in your 40s is working with your changing metabolism instead of against it.

Protein becomes even more important: Aim for 1.2-1.6g per kg of body weight, distributed throughout the day. This helps maintain muscle mass, which is your best defense against a slowing metabolism.

Meal timing matters more: Your body becomes less forgiving of irregular eating patterns. Try to eat at consistent times and avoid skipping meals, which can slow your metabolism further.

Strength training is non-negotiable: While this is a nutrition book, I have to mention that resistance exercise becomes crucial in your 40s to maintain muscle mass and metabolic rate.

Best protein-rich foods for your 40s:

- **Greek yogurt**: High protein, probiotics for gut health
- **Eggs**: Complete protein, choline for brain health
- **Lean fish**: Protein plus omega-3s for inflammation control
- **Legumes**: Protein plus fiber for blood sugar control
- **Quinoa**: Complete plant protein with complex carbs

Priority #2: Control Inflammation

This is the decade when chronic inflammation often begins to develop, setting the stage for future health problems. The good news is that anti-inflammatory foods can dramatically reduce these markers.

Omega-3 fatty acids become crucial: Aim for 1-2 grams of EPA and DHA daily from fish or supplements. Studies show this can reduce inflammation markers by 20-30%.

Antioxidant-rich foods are your friends: Deeply colored fruits and vegetables provide compounds that fight inflammation and protect against cellular damage.

Anti-inflammatory meal template:

- **Base**: Leafy greens or other colorful vegetables
- **Protein**: Fatty fish, organic chicken, or legumes
- **Healthy fat**: Olive oil, avocado, nuts, or seeds
- **Complex carbs**: Quinoa, sweet potato, or wild rice
- **Flavor**: Herbs and spices (especially turmeric, ginger, garlic)

Priority #3: Support Your Changing Hormones

While you can't stop hormonal changes, you can support your body's ability to adapt to them.

For hormone balance:

- **Fiber**: 35-40g daily to help eliminate excess hormones
- **Healthy fats**: 25-30% of calories to support hormone production
- **Phytoestrogens**: Plant compounds that may help balance hormones
- **Stress management**: Since cortisol affects all other hormones

Foods that support hormone balance:

- **Flaxseeds**: 1-2 tablespoons daily for lignans

- **Cruciferous vegetables**: Broccoli, cauliflower, Brussels sprouts
- **Soy foods**: Tofu, tempeh, edamame (if well-tolerated)
- **Healthy fats**: Avocados, olive oil, nuts, fatty fish

Special Considerations for Your 40s

If You're Dealing with Perimenopause:

Women often begin experiencing hormonal fluctuations in their early 40s, even if periods are still regular.

Nutritional support:

- **Iron**: May need less as periods become lighter
- **Calcium**: Increase to 1,200mg daily as bone loss accelerates
- **Vitamin D**: Ensure adequate levels for bone and mood
- **Magnesium**: 400-600mg daily for sleep and mood stability

Foods for perimenopause support:

- **Fatty fish**: For omega-3s and vitamin D
- **Leafy greens**: For calcium, magnesium, and folate
- **Berries**: For antioxidants and fiber
- **Nuts and seeds**: For healthy fats and minerals

If You're a Man Dealing with Declining Testosterone:

Men's testosterone levels begin declining about 1% per year after age 40.

Nutritional support:

- **Zinc**: 15-30mg daily (but not more, as excess can be harmful)
- **Vitamin D**: Maintain optimal levels (40-60 ng/mL)
- **Healthy fats**: Essential for testosterone production
- **Maintain healthy weight**: Excess belly fat increases estrogen

If You're Under High Stress:

Career and family demands often peak in your 40s, which can wreak havoc on your nutrition and health.

Stress-fighting nutrients:

- **B vitamins**: Higher needs during stress periods
- **Magnesium**: Depleted by chronic stress
- **Vitamin C**: Needs increase during stress
- **Adaptogens**: Herbs like ashwagandha may help manage stress response

Practical Strategies That Work

The 40s Meal Formula

Every meal should include:

- **Lean protein**: Palm-sized portion
- **Healthy fat**: Thumb-sized portion
- **Fiber-rich carbs**: Cupped-hand portion

- **Vegetables**: As much as you want

The Energy-Stable Day

- **Upon waking**: Glass of water with lemon
- **Breakfast within 2 hours**: Protein + healthy fat + complex carbs
- **Mid-morning**: Green tea or herbal tea
- **Lunch**: Balanced meal with emphasis on vegetables
- **Afternoon snack**: Protein + healthy fat (if needed)
- **Dinner**: Lighter meal, finished 3 hours before bed

The Weekly Prep Strategy

Spend 1-2 hours on Sunday preparing:

- **Proteins**: Cook chicken, fish, or beans in batches
- **Vegetables**: Wash, chop, and roast a variety
- **Grains**: Cook quinoa, brown rice, or other whole grains
- **Snacks**: Portion out nuts, cut vegetables, make energy balls

Supplements That May Help in Your 40s

While food should always come first, certain supplements can be helpful:

For most people:

- **High-quality multivitamin**: Insurance against nutritional gaps
- **Omega-3 supplement**: If not eating fish 2-3 times per week

- **Vitamin D**: Especially if limited sun exposure
- **Probiotics**: For gut health and immune function

Consider adding:

- **Magnesium**: If dealing with stress, sleep issues, or muscle cramps
- **Coenzyme Q10**: For energy production and heart health
- **Adaptogenic herbs**: For stress management

Warning Signs to Watch For

Seek professional help if you experience:

- Unexplained weight gain despite healthy eating
- Severe fatigue that doesn't improve with rest
- Mood changes, depression, or anxiety
- Sleep problems that persist
- Digestive issues that don't resolve
- Frequent infections or slow healing

The Bottom Line for Your 40s

Your 40s are about adaptation and optimization. Your body is changing, but with the right nutritional approach, these can be some of your best years yet. Focus on supporting your metabolism, controlling inflammation, and working with your hormonal changes rather than against them.

The habits you establish now will carry you into your 50s and beyond feeling strong, energetic, and healthy. This is your time to master the art of eating for your age.

CHAPTER 6
THE PREVENTION YEARS (50S TO 60S) - FIGHTING BACK AGAINST AGE

The Crossroads Decade

Your 50s and 60s represent a crossroads. This is when the gap widens dramatically between people who age successfully and those who struggle with multiple health problems. The exciting news is that you have more control over which path you take than you might think.

I've seen patients in their 70s who have the energy and health of typical 50-year-olds, and I've seen 50-year-olds who seem old beyond their years. The difference usually isn't genetics—it's the accumulated effect of lifestyle choices, with nutrition playing the starring role.

Dr. Luigi Fontana, a researcher at Washington University who studies exceptional aging, puts it this way: "The people who age most successfully are those who make strategic lifestyle changes in their 50s and 60s, before problems become irreversible."

What Makes This Decade Different

The Disease Prevention Window

This is your body's last best chance to prevent chronic diseases or catch them early when they're most treatable. Heart disease, diabetes, osteoporosis, and even some cancers can be largely prevented with the right nutritional approach.

Hormonal Upheaval

For women, menopause brings dramatic hormonal changes that affect everything from bone health to where fat is stored. For men, the gradual decline in testosterone that began in their 40s accelerates, affecting muscle mass, energy, and mood.

The Compound Interest Effect

Good and bad choices from earlier decades start paying significant dividends (or demanding payment) during these years. But here's the hopeful part: positive changes you make now can still have profound effects on your health trajectory.

Your Most Important Health Battles

Battle #1: Keeping Your Heart Strong

Heart disease becomes the leading cause of death starting in your 50s, but it's largely preventable with the right approach.

The Portfolio Diet Approach: Researchers at the University of Toronto developed what they call the "Portfolio Diet"—a combination of foods that can lower cholesterol as effectively as statin medications for some people.

The four components:

1. **Plant sterols**: 2g daily from fortified foods or supplements
2. **Viscous fiber**: 10-15g daily from oats, barley, and psyllium
3. **Soy protein**: 25g daily replacing animal protein
4. **Tree nuts**: 45g (about 1.5 ounces) daily

Heart-healthy daily menu example:

- **Breakfast**: Oatmeal with ground flaxseed and berries, soy milk
- **Lunch**: Large salad with beans, avocado, and olive oil dressing
- **Snack**: Small handful of almonds
- **Dinner**: Baked tofu or salmon with steamed broccoli and quinoa

Battle #2: Preventing Diabetes

Type 2 diabetes affects 26% of adults over 65, but it's largely preventable with targeted nutrition changes.

The Finnish Diabetes Prevention Study followed 522 people at high risk for diabetes for four years. Those who made specific dietary changes reduced their diabetes risk by 58%—better results than medication.

The key changes:

- **Weight loss**: Even 5-7% reduction significantly lowers risk
- **Fiber increase**: 35-40g daily from whole foods
- **Healthy fats**: Focus on monounsaturated and omega-3 fats

- **Portion control**: Using smaller plates and measuring portions
- **Regular meal timing**: Helps stabilize blood sugar

Blood sugar-friendly plate method:

- **1/2 plate**: Non-starchy vegetables
- **1/4 plate**: Lean protein
- **1/4 plate**: Complex carbohydrates
- **Add**: Healthy fat (olive oil, nuts, avocado)

Battle #3: Protecting Your Bones

Bone loss accelerates significantly after menopause for women and after age 65 for men. But proper nutrition can slow or even reverse this process.

Beyond calcium: While calcium is important, bone health requires a team of nutrients working together.

The bone health dream team:

- **Calcium**: 1,200mg daily for women over 50, men over 70
- **Vitamin D**: 800-1,000 IU daily, more if deficient
- **Vitamin K2**: 200-300mcg daily for calcium utilization
- **Magnesium**: 400-500mg daily
- **Protein**: 1.2-1.6g per kg body weight

Bone-building foods:

- **Dairy products**: If well-tolerated

- **Leafy greens**: Kale, collards, bok choy
- **Canned fish with bones**: Sardines, salmon
- **Almonds and sesame seeds**: Plant calcium sources
- **Fortified plant milks**: If avoiding dairy

Battle #4: Keeping Your Brain Sharp

Cognitive decline isn't inevitable. The MIND diet (Mediterranean-DASH Intervention for Neurodegenerative Delay) can reduce Alzheimer's risk by up to 53%.

Brain-boosting foods to emphasize:

- **Leafy greens**: At least 6 servings per week
- **Berries**: 2+ servings per week, especially blueberries
- **Nuts**: 5+ servings per week
- **Fish**: At least once per week
- **Beans**: 3+ servings per week
- **Whole grains**: 3+ servings per day

Brain-damaging foods to limit:

- **Red meat**: Less than 4 servings per week
- **Butter and margarine**: Less than 1 tablespoon daily
- **Cheese**: Less than 1 serving per week
- **Fried foods**: Less than 1 serving per week
- **Sweets**: Less than 5 servings per week

Navigating Menopause with Nutrition

The Hormone Replacement Debate

While hormone replacement therapy can be helpful for some women, nutrition can significantly ease menopausal symptoms for many.

Natural approaches for hot flashes:

- **Soy isoflavones**: 50-100mg daily may reduce hot flashes by 40-50%
- **Flaxseeds**: 2 tablespoons ground daily for lignans
- **Black cohosh**: Herbal supplement that may help some women

Weight management during menopause:

The average woman gains 10-15 pounds during menopause, but this isn't inevitable.

Strategies that work:

- **Increase protein**: To 1.2-1.6g per kg body weight to maintain muscle
- **Time carbohydrates**: Eat them earlier in the day when insulin sensitivity is higher
- **Include strength training**: Essential for maintaining muscle mass
- **Manage stress**: High cortisol worsens menopause symptoms

Special Considerations for Men

Supporting Healthy Testosterone

While testosterone naturally declines with age, nutrition can help maintain healthy levels.

Testosterone-supporting strategies:

- **Maintain healthy weight**: Excess belly fat converts testosterone to estrogen
- **Include zinc-rich foods**: Oysters, lean meat, pumpkin seeds
- **Get adequate vitamin D**: Low levels correlate with low testosterone
- **Don't restrict fats too severely**: Testosterone is made from cholesterol

Prostate Health

Prostate problems affect most men over 50, but nutrition can help.

Prostate-protective foods:

- **Tomatoes**: Rich in lycopene, especially when cooked
- **Green tea**: Contains compounds that may protect prostate cells
- **Cruciferous vegetables**: May help process hormones more effectively
- **Omega-3 fatty acids**: Anti-inflammatory effects may benefit prostate health

Age-Specific Supplement Considerations

For most people in their 50s and 60s:

- **Comprehensive multivitamin**: To cover nutritional gaps
- **Omega-3 supplement**: 1-2g daily of EPA and DHA
- **Vitamin D**: 1,000-2,000 IU daily, depending on blood levels
- **Probiotics**: For gut health and immune function

Consider adding:

- **Coenzyme Q10**: 100-200mg daily for heart and energy support
- **Magnesium**: 400-600mg daily for bone health and sleep
- **Vitamin K2**: 200-300mcg daily for bone and heart health

For women post-menopause:

- **Calcium**: If not getting enough from food
- **Additional vitamin D**: Higher needs for bone health

For men over 50:

- **Lycopene**: If not eating tomatoes regularly
- **Saw palmetto**: May support prostate health (consult your doctor first)

The Power of Meal Timing

Why when you eat matters more now:

Your body's ability to handle large meals and irregular eating patterns decreases with age. Strategic meal timing can improve:

- Blood sugar control

- Weight management
- Sleep quality
- Energy levels

Optimal eating schedule:

- **Breakfast**: Within 2 hours of waking, protein-rich
- **Lunch**: Largest meal of the day when insulin sensitivity is highest
- **Dinner**: Lighter meal, finished 3 hours before bedtime
- **Snacks**: If needed, combine protein with healthy fat

Creating Your Prevention Plan

Week 1-2: Foundation Building

- Track what you currently eat to identify problem areas
- Add one serving of vegetables to each meal
- Replace refined grains with whole grains
- Include protein at every meal

Week 3-4: Anti-Inflammatory Focus

- Add fatty fish twice per week
- Include berries daily
- Use olive oil as your primary fat
- Add anti-inflammatory spices (turmeric, ginger, garlic)

Week 5-6: Optimization

- Fine-tune portion sizes

- Address any remaining processed foods
- Add targeted supplements if needed
- Focus on meal timing

Week 7-8: Personalization

- Adjust based on how you feel
- Address specific health concerns
- Work with healthcare providers as needed
- Plan for long-term sustainability

The Bottom Line for Your 50s and 60s

This is your prevention decade. The choices you make now will largely determine your health trajectory for the next 20-30 years. The good news is that it's not too late to make dramatic improvements in your health, and the changes you make now can have profound effects on how you age.

Focus on the big picture: prevent chronic disease, maintain muscle and bone mass, keep your brain sharp, and optimize your energy. With the right nutritional approach, your 70s and 80s can be active, healthy, and fulfilling decades.

CHAPTER 7
THE WISDOM YEARS (70S AND BEYOND) - STAYING STRONG AND SHARP

Redefining What It Means to Age

Let me tell you about Eleanor, one of my favorite patients. She's 87 years old, lives independently, travels internationally, volunteers at three different organizations, and has more energy than many of my 50-year-old patients. When people ask her secret, she says, "I eat like my life depends on it—because it does."

Eleanor represents what researchers call "successful aging"—maintaining physical function, cognitive ability, and independence well into advanced years. And contrary to popular belief, this isn't primarily about good genetics. It's about smart choices, with nutrition playing the lead role.

The exciting research coming out of places like Harvard's Study of Adult Development (which has followed people for over 80 years) shows that how you age is much more under your control than most people realize. The people who thrive in their 80s and 90s aren't necessarily those who had the best genes—they're those who made the best choices throughout their lives, especially regarding nutrition.

The Unique Challenges and Opportunities of This Life Stage

The Challenge: Multiple Changes Happening at Once

Your 70s and beyond bring a perfect storm of changes that can affect nutrition:

- **Appetite changes**: Many people eat less due to altered taste and smell

- **Medication effects**: Multiple prescriptions can affect nutrient absorption
- **Social factors**: Cooking for one, limited mobility, or social isolation
- **Physical changes**: Dental problems, swallowing difficulties, or arthritis
- **Cognitive changes**: Memory issues that might affect meal planning

The Opportunity: More Time and Motivation

But this life stage also offers unique advantages:

- **More time**: To focus on health and meal preparation
- **Accumulated wisdom**: Better understanding of what works for your body
- **Strong motivation**: Awareness that health choices directly impact quality of life
- **Fewer external pressures**: Less influenced by work schedules or social expectations

Your New Nutritional Priorities

Priority #1: Maintaining Muscle Mass and Strength

Muscle loss accelerates significantly after age 70, but proper nutrition can slow or even reverse this process. Research shows that well-nourished older adults can maintain muscle function equivalent to people 20 years younger.

Protein becomes absolutely critical: Adults over 70 need significantly more protein than younger people—1.6-2.0g per kg of body weight daily.

Why protein requirements increase:

- Older muscles are less responsive to protein intake
- Absorption of amino acids decreases
- Muscle protein breakdown increases
- Recovery from illness requires extra protein

High-quality protein sources for seniors:

- **Eggs**: Easy to digest, complete protein
- **Greek yogurt**: High protein plus probiotics
- **Fish**: Easily digestible protein plus omega-3s
- **Protein powder**: Convenient way to boost intake
- **Beans and lentils**: Plant protein plus fiber

The 30-gram rule: Try to include at least 30g of high-quality protein at each meal to maximize muscle protein synthesis.

Priority #2: Supporting Brain Health and Cognitive Function

While some cognitive changes are normal with aging, severe cognitive decline isn't inevitable. Nutrition can significantly influence brain health and may help prevent dementia.

The MIND diet results: People who followed the MIND diet closely had cognitive function equivalent to being 7.5 years younger than those who didn't.

Brain-protecting nutrients:

- **Omega-3 fatty acids**: Especially DHA for brain structure
- **Antioxidants**: To protect brain cells from damage
- **B vitamins**: For nerve function and neurotransmitter production
- **Vitamin D**: Low levels linked to cognitive decline

Daily brain-healthy eating pattern:

- **Breakfast**: Oatmeal with blueberries and walnuts
- **Lunch**: Spinach salad with salmon and olive oil dressing
- **Snack**: Green tea and a small handful of nuts
- **Dinner**: Lentil soup with vegetables and whole grain bread

Priority #3: Preventing Malnutrition

Malnutrition affects up to 50% of hospitalized older adults and is a major risk factor for falls, infections, and loss of independence.

Warning signs of malnutrition:

- Unintentional weight loss
- Fatigue or weakness
- Frequent infections
- Slow wound healing
- Depression or confusion

Strategies to maintain adequate nutrition:

- **Eat frequently**: 5-6 small meals may be easier than 3 large ones
- **Enhance flavors**: Use herbs, spices, and seasonings liberally
- **Make calories count**: Choose nutrient-dense foods
- **Stay social**: Eat with others when possible
- **Get help**: Don't be too proud to accept assistance with shopping or cooking

Working with Age-Related Changes

When Appetite Decreases

Many older adults find they're just not as hungry as they used to be. This is partly due to changes in hormones that regulate appetite and partly due to decreased activity levels.

Strategies to stimulate appetite:

- **Exercise**: Even light physical activity can increase hunger
- **Eat with others**: Social meals are more appealing
- **Enhance aromas**: The smell of food cooking can stimulate appetite
- **Try new foods**: Novel flavors can be more appealing than familiar ones
- **Time medications carefully**: Some medications are better taken after meals

When Taste and Smell Change

Loss of taste and smell is common with aging and can make food seem less appealing.

Flavor enhancement strategies:

- **Use more seasonings**: Herbs, spices, lemon juice, vinegar
- **Try temperature contrasts**: Cold foods with warm foods
- **Enhance colors**: Colorful foods are more appealing
- **Experiment with textures**: Crunchy additions to soft foods
- **Focus on umami**: Mushrooms, aged cheeses, tomatoes provide savory flavor

When Chewing Becomes Difficult

Dental problems or poorly fitting dentures can make eating challenging.

Texture modifications:

- **Soft proteins**: Eggs, fish, ground meat, beans
- **Cooked vegetables**: Steamed, roasted, or pureed
- **Smoothies**: Blend fruits, vegetables, protein powder, and healthy fats
- **Soups and stews**: Nutrient-dense and easy to eat
- **Nut butters**: Instead of whole nuts

Special Nutritional Needs for Seniors

Vitamin B12 Becomes Critical

Up to 30% of adults over 70 have difficulty absorbing vitamin B12 from food due to decreased stomach acid production.

Signs of B12 deficiency:

- Fatigue and weakness
- Memory problems
- Balance issues
- Tingling in hands or feet

B12 solutions:

- **Sublingual supplements**: Absorbed under the tongue
- **Fortified foods**: Cereals, nutritional yeast
- **B12 injections**: If absorption is severely impaired

Vitamin D Requirements Increase

Older adults need more vitamin D due to:

- Less efficient skin production
- Reduced kidney function
- Less time outdoors
- Decreased absorption

Vitamin D targets for seniors:

- **Blood level**: 30-50 ng/mL (optimal range)
- **Daily intake**: 1,000-2,000 IU (may need more if deficient)
- **Food sources**: Fatty fish, fortified foods, egg yolks
- **Safe sun exposure**: 15-20 minutes daily when possible

Calcium and Bone Health

Fracture risk increases significantly with age, making bone health crucial for maintaining independence.

Calcium absorption tips:

- **Take with food**: Improves absorption
- **Split doses**: No more than 500mg at once
- **Include vitamin D**: Essential for calcium absorption
- **Don't exceed 2,000mg daily**: Higher amounts may increase heart disease risk

Hydration Becomes More Critical

Dehydration is a serious risk for older adults due to:

- Decreased thirst sensation
- Kidney changes
- Medication effects
- Fear of bathroom urgency

Daily hydration goals:

- **6-8 glasses**: Of fluid daily (water, tea, soup, etc.)
- **Monitor urine color**: Pale yellow indicates good hydration
- **Eat water-rich foods**: Fruits, vegetables, soups
- **Limit alcohol and caffeine**: Can contribute to dehydration

Supplements That May Be Helpful

Generally recommended for seniors:

- **Vitamin B12**: 25-100mcg daily
- **Vitamin D**: 1,000-2,000 IU daily
- **Omega-3 fatty acids**: 1-2g daily of EPA and DHA

- **Probiotics**: For gut health and immune function

Consider with healthcare provider:

- **Calcium**: If dietary intake is inadequate
- **Magnesium**: For muscle function and bone health
- **Protein powder**: If struggling to meet protein needs
- **Multivitamin**: As insurance against nutritional gaps

Meal Planning for Independence

The Simple Meal Formula

Every meal should include:

- **High-quality protein**: 25-30g
- **Colorful vegetables**: 1-2 servings
- **Healthy fat**: 1-2 servings
- **Complex carbohydrate**: 1 serving (optional)

Easy meal ideas:

Breakfast options:

- Greek yogurt with berries and granola
- Scrambled eggs with spinach and whole grain toast
- Protein smoothie with banana and peanut butter
- Oatmeal with protein powder and nuts

Lunch options:

- Tuna salad on whole grain bread with tomato
- Lentil soup with whole grain crackers
- Chicken salad with mixed greens
- Egg salad sandwich with avocado

Dinner options:

- Baked fish with roasted vegetables
- Slow cooker chicken and vegetables
- Bean and vegetable soup
- Omelet with vegetables and cheese

Working with Healthcare Providers

When to seek help:

- Unintentional weight loss of more than 5% in 6 months
- Difficulty eating or swallowing
- Loss of appetite lasting more than a few days
- Signs of nutrient deficiency
- Changes in cognitive function

Questions to ask your healthcare provider:

- Are any of my medications affecting my appetite or nutrition?
- Should I be taking any specific supplements?
- Do I need any nutritional blood tests?
- Are there community resources available to help with meals?

The Social Aspect of Eating

Combating isolation:

- **Community meal programs**: Many areas offer senior dining programs
- **Cooking clubs**: Share meal preparation with friends or neighbors
- **Family meals**: Regular dinners with family or friends
- **Meal delivery services**: Some offer social interaction along with meals

The Bottom Line for Your 70s and Beyond

Nutrition in your senior years isn't just about preventing disease—it's about maintaining independence, energy, and quality of life. The goal is to age successfully, staying strong and sharp for as long as possible.

Focus on nutrient-dense foods, adequate protein, brain-healthy choices, and maintaining the joy of eating. With the right approach, these can be some of your most fulfilling and healthy years yet.

Remember Eleanor's philosophy: eat like your life depends on it, because it does. Your nutritional choices at this stage directly impact your ability to live independently, stay mentally sharp, and enjoy life to the fullest.

CHAPTER 8
SPECIAL SITUATIONS - WHEN LIFE THROWS YOU CURVEBALLS

When Standard Advice Isn't Enough

Throughout this book, I've given you age-based nutritional guidance that works for most people. But life doesn't always follow standard patterns. Sometimes health conditions, medications, lifestyle factors, or genetic variations mean you need a modified approach.

This chapter addresses those situations when you might need to adapt the general recommendations to fit your specific circumstances.

Managing Chronic Conditions at Any Age

Type 2 Diabetes: Eating to Control Blood Sugar

Diabetes affects people of all ages, but the nutritional approach needs to be adjusted based on your life stage.

Core principles for all ages:

- **Consistent carbohydrate intake**: Same amount at each meal
- **Protein at every meal**: Helps stabilize blood sugar
- **High-fiber foods**: Slow glucose absorption
- **Healthy fats**: Don't affect blood sugar directly

Age-specific modifications:

20s-40s with diabetes:

- Focus on building healthy habits for life
- Learn carbohydrate counting
- Emphasize weight management if needed
- Plan for pregnancy (women) with tight glucose control

50s-60s with diabetes:

- Screen for diabetes complications
- Adjust for other health conditions
- Monitor for medication interactions
- Focus on heart disease prevention

70s+ with diabetes:

- Prevent hypoglycemia (low blood sugar)
- Maintain adequate nutrition
- Adjust targets for quality of life
- Monitor for medication side effects

Heart Disease: Protecting Your Cardiovascular System

The therapeutic lifestyle changes (TLC) approach:

- **Saturated fat**: Less than 7% of total calories
- **Cholesterol**: Less than 200mg daily
- **Sodium**: Less than 2,300mg daily (ideally 1,500mg)
- **Fiber**: 25-35g daily from whole foods

Heart-healthy meal pattern:

- **Breakfast**: Oatmeal with berries and ground flaxseed
- **Lunch**: Lentil soup with whole grain bread
- **Snack**: Apple with almond butter
- **Dinner**: Baked fish, steamed broccoli, quinoa

Osteoporosis: Building and Maintaining Strong Bones

Beyond calcium: Bone health requires multiple nutrients working together.

The bone health protocol:

- **Calcium**: 1,000-1,200mg daily from food and supplements
- **Vitamin D**: 800-1,000 IU daily (more if deficient)
- **Vitamin K2**: 180-200mcg daily
- **Magnesium**: 400-500mg daily
- **Protein**: 1.2-1.6g per kg body weight

Bone-building foods:

- **Dairy products**: If well-tolerated
- **Leafy greens**: Especially kale and collards
- **Canned fish with bones**: Sardines, salmon
- **Fortified plant milks**: Calcium and vitamin D
- **Sesame seeds**: High in calcium

Medication and Supplement Interactions

Common medications that affect nutrition:

Blood thinners (warfarin):

- **Vitamin K interaction**: Maintain consistent intake of leafy greens
- **Avoid high-dose vitamin E**: Can increase bleeding risk
- **Limit alcohol**: Affects medication effectiveness

Acid-blocking medications (PPIs, H2 blockers):

- **Vitamin B12**: Reduced absorption due to decreased stomach acid
- **Iron**: Better absorbed with vitamin C
- **Calcium**: Choose calcium citrate over calcium carbonate

Diabetes medications:

- **Metformin**: Can deplete vitamin B12 and folate
- **Insulin**: Timing with meals becomes crucial
- **Monitor for hypoglycemia**: Especially if meal timing changes

Cholesterol medications (statins):

- **Coenzyme Q10**: May be depleted; consider supplementation
- **Grapefruit**: Can increase medication levels (avoid or limit)
- **Alcohol**: Limit to reduce liver stress

Dietary Restrictions and Special Diets

Vegetarian and Vegan Nutrition by Age

Plant-based eating at different life stages:

Younger adults (20s-40s):

- **Iron**: Combine with vitamin C foods for absorption
- **Vitamin B12**: Essential supplement (2.4mcg daily minimum)
- **Protein**: Combine complementary proteins throughout the day
- **Omega-3s**: Algae-based supplements for DHA and EPA

Middle age (50s-60s):

- **Increased protein needs**: 1.2-1.6g per kg body weight
- **Calcium**: From fortified foods or supplements
- **Vitamin D**: Often need supplements regardless of diet
- **Zinc**: May need attention, especially for men

Seniors (70s+):

- **Protein adequacy**: May need protein powder or bars
- **Vitamin B12**: Higher needs and absorption issues
- **Calorie density**: Plant foods are often lower in calories
- **Social support**: Help with meal planning and preparation

Gluten-Free Nutrition

Whether due to celiac disease or non-celiac gluten sensitivity, going gluten-free requires careful planning.

Nutritional concerns:

- **Fiber**: Many gluten-free products are lower in fiber
- **B vitamins**: Fortified wheat products are a major source
- **Iron**: Enriched wheat products provide significant iron
- **Cost and convenience**: Gluten-free options are often more expensive

Healthy gluten-free strategies:

- **Focus on naturally gluten-free foods**: Fruits, vegetables, lean proteins
- **Choose whole grain alternatives**: Quinoa, brown rice, millet
- **Read labels carefully**: Hidden gluten in processed foods
- **Consider supplements**: B vitamins, iron if needed

Food Allergies and Intolerances

Lactose Intolerance

Affects up to 65% of adults worldwide, with prevalence increasing with age.

Alternatives to dairy:

- **Lactose-free dairy products**: Milk, yogurt, cheese
- **Fortified plant milks**: Soy, almond, oat, pea protein
- **Calcium-rich foods**: Leafy greens, canned fish with bones, tahini
- **Lactase supplements**: Can help digest lactose-containing foods

Food Allergies in Adults

Adult-onset food allergies are becoming more common.

Common adult food allergies:

- **Shellfish**: Most common adult food allergy
- **Tree nuts**: Can develop at any age
- **Fish**: Sometimes develops after being able to eat fish previously
- **Soy**: May develop in adulthood

Managing food allergies:

- **Read labels carefully**: Allergens must be clearly labeled
- **Carry emergency medication**: If prescribed by your doctor
- **Work with a dietitian**: To ensure nutritional adequacy
- **Find substitutes**: For allergenic foods in your usual diet

Digestive Issues and Gut Health

Irritable Bowel Syndrome (IBS)

IBS affects 10-15% of adults and can significantly impact nutrition.

The low-FODMAP approach: A diet low in fermentable carbohydrates can reduce IBS symptoms in 70% of people.

High-FODMAP foods to limit:

- **Fruits**: Apples, pears, stone fruits

- **Vegetables**: Onions, garlic, asparagus
- **Legumes**: Beans, lentils, chickpeas
- **Grains**: Wheat, rye, barley
- **Dairy**: Milk, soft cheeses

Low-FODMAP alternatives:

- **Fruits**: Berries, citrus, grapes
- **Vegetables**: Carrots, peppers, spinach
- **Proteins**: All meats, fish, eggs
- **Grains**: Rice, oats, quinoa

Inflammatory Bowel Disease (IBD)

Crohn's disease and ulcerative colitis require specialized nutritional management.

During flares:

- **Easy-to-digest foods**: White rice, lean proteins, cooked vegetables
- **Avoid high-fiber foods**: Can worsen symptoms during flares
- **Small, frequent meals**: Easier on the digestive system
- **Adequate hydration**: Important for healing

During remission:

- **Anti-inflammatory foods**: Omega-3 rich fish, colorful vegetables
- **Probiotic foods**: May help maintain remission

- **Adequate calories**: To support healing and prevent weight loss
- **Monitor trigger foods**: Keep a food diary

Eating Disorders and Disordered Eating

Recovery Nutrition

Eating disorder recovery requires specialized care, but general principles include:

Mechanical eating: Regular meals and snacks regardless of hunger **All foods fit**: No "good" or "bad" foods **Weight restoration**: If needed for health **Professional support**: Registered dietitians specialized in eating disorders

Disordered Eating in Older Adults

Often overlooked, disordered eating can affect seniors.

Risk factors:

- Social isolation
- Depression
- Medication effects
- Financial constraints
- Physical limitations

Warning signs:

- Significant weight loss

- Avoiding social meals
- Extreme food restrictions
- Preoccupation with weight

Economic Constraints

Eating Well on a Budget

Good nutrition doesn't have to be expensive, but it does require planning.

Budget-friendly nutritious foods:

- **Dried beans and lentils**: Cheapest protein source
- **Eggs**: Inexpensive complete protein
- **Canned fish**: Affordable omega-3 source
- **Frozen vegetables**: As nutritious as fresh, often cheaper
- **Whole grains in bulk**: Oats, brown rice, quinoa

Money-saving strategies:

- **Meal planning**: Reduces food waste and impulse purchases
- **Batch cooking**: Saves time and money
- **Seasonal produce**: Usually cheaper and more nutritious
- **Store brands**: Often just as good as name brands
- **Community resources**: Food banks, senior meal programs

The Bottom Line on Special Situations

While the age-based recommendations in this book provide a solid foundation, life sometimes requires modifications. The key is working with qualified healthcare providers—doctors, registered dietitians, and other specialists—to develop an approach that meets your specific needs while still following the basic principles of eating for your age.

Don't let special circumstances become an excuse to abandon healthy eating altogether. Instead, view them as opportunities to fine-tune your approach and develop an even more personalized nutrition plan.

Remember: there's almost always a way to eat well, regardless of your circumstances. It might require creativity, flexibility, and professional help, but it's worth the effort. Your health—at any age—depends on it.

CHAPTER 9
MAKING IT WORK - PRACTICAL TIPS FOR EVERY AGE

From Knowledge to Action

You now understand why your nutritional needs change with age and what you should be eating at different life stages. But knowing what to do and actually doing it are two different things. This chapter bridges that gap with practical strategies that make healthy eating achievable, sustainable, and enjoyable at any age.

The Foundation: Building Habits That Stick

Start Small, Think Big

The biggest mistake people make when trying to improve their nutrition is attempting to change everything at once. Research from Stanford University shows that people who make one small change at a time are 40% more likely to maintain their new habits long-term compared to those who try to overhaul their entire diet.

The 1% principle: Aim to improve your eating by just 1% each day. These tiny improvements compound over time into dramatic results.

Examples of 1% improvements:

- Add one extra serving of vegetables to your day
- Replace one processed snack with a whole food option

- Drink one extra glass of water
- Take three deep breaths before each meal
- Eat one meal without distractions

Age-Specific Implementation Strategies

For Your 20s and 30s: Building the Foundation

Challenge: Busy schedules, limited cooking experience, social pressures

The Prep-Ahead Strategy

Sunday meal prep becomes your secret weapon:

Spend 2 hours on Sunday:

- **Proteins**: Cook chicken breasts, hard-boil eggs, cook a pot of beans
- **Vegetables**: Wash and chop raw veggies, roast a big batch of mixed vegetables
- **Grains**: Cook quinoa, brown rice, or other whole grains
- **Snacks**: Portion out nuts, cut up fruits, make energy balls

The 5-Minute Meal Formula Every meal should be assemblable in 5 minutes or less:

- **Base**: Pre-cooked grain or leafy greens
- **Protein**: Pre-cooked protein or quick options like eggs or Greek yogurt
- **Vegetables**: Pre-cut fresh or pre-roasted vegetables

- **Fat**: Avocado, nuts, olive oil, or tahini
- **Flavor**: Herbs, spices, lemon juice, or healthy dressing

Social Eating Strategies

- **Restaurant tactics**: Look up menus in advance, ask for modifications
- **Party planning**: Eat a protein-rich snack before going out
- **Alcohol management**: Alternate alcoholic drinks with water, eat before drinking

For Your 40s: Adapting to Change

Challenge: Slowing metabolism, increasing responsibilities, hormonal changes

The Metabolic Reset Protocol

Week 1-2: Stabilize blood sugar

- Eat protein at every meal and snack
- Choose complex carbohydrates over simple ones
- Avoid skipping meals
- Limit added sugars to less than 25g daily

Week 3-4: Optimize meal timing

- Eat your largest meal earlier in the day
- Stop eating 3 hours before bedtime
- Consider a 12-hour overnight fast (8 PM to 8 AM)
- Space meals 4-5 hours apart

Week 5-6: Focus on inflammation control

- Include omega-3 rich foods daily
- Eat at least 5 servings of colorful vegetables
- Add anti-inflammatory spices (turmeric, ginger, garlic)
- Limit processed foods and refined oils

The Stress-Eating Solution

Stress eating often peaks during the 40s due to career and family pressures.

Create stress-eating alternatives:

- **Physical**: Take a walk, do jumping jacks, stretch
- **Mental**: Practice deep breathing, call a friend, listen to music
- **Nutritional**: Keep healthy snacks visible, prepare stress-eating alternatives

Healthy stress-eating options:

- Dark chocolate (70% cacao or higher)
- Trail mix with nuts and dried fruit
- Greek yogurt with berries
- Herbal tea with a small piece of cheese

For Your 50s and 60s: Prevention and Optimization

Challenge: Chronic disease prevention, hormonal changes, medication interactions

The Prevention-Focused Meal Plan

Daily template:

- **Breakfast**: High-protein, anti-inflammatory
- **Lunch**: Largest meal, balanced macronutrients
- **Dinner**: Lighter, early timing
- **Snacks**: If needed, protein + healthy fat

Sample prevention-focused day:

Breakfast (7:00 AM):

- 2 eggs scrambled with spinach
- 1 slice whole grain toast with avocado
- 1 cup berries
- Green tea

Lunch (12:00 PM):

- Large salad with mixed greens, grilled salmon, chickpeas, olive oil dressing
- 1 small sweet potato
- Sparkling water with lemon

Snack (3:00 PM, if needed):

- Small handful of almonds
- 1 small apple

Dinner (6:00 PM):

- 4 oz grilled chicken
- Steamed broccoli with lemon
- 1/2 cup quinoa
- Herbal tea

The Supplement Schedule

If you're taking supplements, timing matters:

With breakfast:

- Multivitamin (better absorption with food)
- Vitamin D (fat-soluble, better with meals)
- Omega-3s (reduce fishy aftertaste)

With dinner:

- Magnesium (may promote relaxation)
- Probiotics (if recommended with food)

Before bed:

- Any sleep-supporting supplements

For Your 70s and Beyond: Maintaining Independence

Challenge: Decreased appetite, medication interactions, social isolation

The Independence-Preservation Plan

Make every bite count:

- Choose nutrient-dense foods over empty calories
- Add protein powder to smoothies, soups, or oatmeal
- Use healthy fats liberally to increase calories
- Enhance flavors with herbs and spices

The Senior-Friendly Kitchen Setup

Easy-access organization:

- Keep frequently used items at counter height
- Store healthy snacks at eye level
- Pre-portion nuts, dried fruits, and other snacks
- Keep a pitcher of water visible as a hydration reminder

Simple cooking strategies:

- **One-pot meals**: Soups, stews, casseroles
- **Slow cooker**: Set it and forget it cooking
- **Pre-cut vegetables**: Save energy and time
- **Protein shortcuts**: Rotisserie chicken, canned fish, eggs

Universal Strategies for All Ages

The Hydration Habit

Dehydration affects people of all ages but becomes more dangerous as we get older.

Hydration strategies:

- **Start your day with water**: Keep a glass by your bedside
- **Use visual cues**: Rubber bands on your water bottle to track intake
- **Flavor your water**: Add lemon, cucumber, mint, or berries
- **Eat your water**: Include water-rich foods like soup, fruits, and vegetables

The Mindful Eating Practice

Eating mindfully becomes more important with age as our natural hunger and fullness cues can become less reliable.

Basic mindful eating steps:

1. **Before eating**: Take three deep breaths and check in with your hunger level
2. **During eating**: Eat slowly, chew thoroughly, put your fork down between bites
3. **After eating**: Check in with your fullness level and satisfaction

The Social Connection

Eating with others improves both nutrition and overall wellbeing at any age.

Ways to eat socially:

- **Family meals**: Even if it's just once a week
- **Cooking together**: Involve family or friends in meal preparation

- **Community meals**: Join senior centers, religious groups, or community organizations
- **Virtual meals**: Video calls with family or friends during meals

Troubleshooting Common Problems

"I don't have time to cook"

Time-saving solutions:

- **Batch cooking**: Cook once, eat multiple times
- **Simple meals**: Focus on 3-5 ingredient recipes
- **Kitchen shortcuts**: Pre-cut vegetables, rotisserie chicken, frozen fruits
- **One-pan meals**: Minimal cleanup required

"Healthy food is too expensive"

Budget-friendly strategies:

- **Buy in season**: Cheaper and more nutritious
- **Frozen is fine**: Often less expensive than fresh
- **Plant proteins**: Beans and lentils are cheaper than meat
- **Buy in bulk**: Nuts, seeds, grains, and legumes

"I don't like vegetables"

Vegetable acceptance strategies:

- **Start small**: Add tiny amounts to familiar foods

- **Try different preparations**: Roasted, sautéed, pureed into sauces
- **Pair with favorites**: Add vegetables to pizza, pasta, or sandwiches
- **Smoothies**: Blend spinach or kale into fruit smoothies

"I eat out too much"

Restaurant success strategies:

- **Research menus ahead**: Many restaurants post nutrition information online
- **Ask for modifications**: Most restaurants will accommodate reasonable requests
- **Control portions**: Ask for a to-go box at the beginning of the meal
- **Focus on protein and vegetables**: These are usually the safest bets

Creating Your Personal Action Plan

Step 1: Assess Your Current Situation

- What age-specific recommendations apply to you?
- What are your biggest nutritional challenges?
- What resources do you have available (time, money, cooking skills)?
- What health conditions or medications do you need to consider?

Step 2: Set SMART Goals Make your goals Specific, Measurable, Achievable, Relevant, and Time-bound.

Examples of SMART nutrition goals:

- "I will eat 5 servings of fruits and vegetables every day for the next month"
- "I will include 25g of protein at breakfast 5 days per week"
- "I will meal prep for 2 hours every Sunday for the next 8 weeks"

Step 3: Start with One Change Choose the one change that will have the biggest impact on your health and start there.

High-impact changes by age:

- **20s-30s**: Establish regular meal timing
- **40s**: Add anti-inflammatory foods daily
- **50s-60s**: Increase protein intake
- **70s+**: Focus on nutrient density

Step 4: Plan for Obstacles What barriers are likely to get in your way? How will you overcome them?

Common obstacles and solutions:

- **Busy schedule**: Prep meals in advance
- **Social pressure**: Have a plan for social eating situations
- **Lack of motivation**: Find an accountability partner
- **All-or-nothing thinking**: Remember that progress, not perfection, is the goal

Step 5: Track Your Progress Keep a simple food diary or use a smartphone app to monitor your changes.

What to track:

- Meals and snacks
- Energy levels
- Sleep quality
- Mood
- Any symptoms

Step 6: Adjust as Needed Your plan should evolve as you learn what works for your body and lifestyle.

The Bottom Line: Making It Sustainable

The best nutrition plan is the one you can follow consistently over time. Don't try to be perfect—try to be consistent. Small improvements maintained over months and years will have a much bigger impact on your health than dramatic changes that only last a few weeks.

Remember: you're not just changing how you eat for a few months. You're developing a way of eating that will support your health and vitality for the rest of your life. Take your time, be patient with yourself, and celebrate small victories along the way.

Your future self will thank you for every healthy choice you make today.

CONCLUSION
YOUR JOURNEY TO AGELESS VITALITY

As we reach the end of this journey together, I want you to think about what drew you to this book in the first place. Maybe you picked it up because you've noticed changes in how your body responds to food. Maybe you're dealing with a health concern and want to take control through nutrition. Or maybe you simply want to age as well as possible and are looking for a roadmap.

Whatever brought you here, I hope you're leaving with something more valuable than just information—I hope you're leaving with a new perspective on what it means to eat for your age and age successfully.

The Big Picture

Throughout this book, we've explored how your nutritional needs change across the decades of your life. We've seen how the foundational choices you make in your 20s and 30s set the stage for how you'll age. We've discovered how the metabolic shifts of your 40s require new strategies for maintaining health and energy. We've learned how the prevention-focused approach of your 50s and 60s can dramatically influence your disease risk. And we've seen how the wisdom years of your 70s and beyond can be some of your most vibrant if you provide your body with what it needs.

But beyond all the specific recommendations and scientific research, there's a simpler truth at the heart of this book: **your age is not your fate.**

Yes, your body changes as you age. Yes, you need to adapt your nutritional approach accordingly. But aging successfully isn't about luck or genetics—it's about making informed choices that support your body's changing needs throughout your life.

The Three Pillars of Ageless Eating

As you move forward, remember these three fundamental principles that apply at every age:

1. Nutrition Density Becomes More Important Over Time

As your calorie needs decrease with age, every bite becomes more important. This doesn't mean eating less—it means eating smarter. Choose foods that provide the most nutrition per calorie: colorful vegetables, lean proteins, healthy fats, and whole grains.

2. Protein Is Your Friend at Every Age

Contrary to outdated advice, your protein needs don't decrease as you age—they actually increase. Protein is essential for maintaining muscle mass, supporting immune function, and preserving independence as you age.

3. Consistency Trumps Perfection

You don't need to eat perfectly to age well. You need to eat consistently well. Small, sustainable changes maintained over time will have a much bigger impact on your health than dramatic changes that only last a few weeks.

Looking Forward: Your Next Steps

Now that you understand the principles of eating for your age, here's how to put them into practice:

Start Where You Are

Look at the recommendations for your current age group and identify the one change that would have the biggest impact on your health. Maybe it's adding more protein to your breakfast, including more anti-inflammatory foods in your diet, or simply eating more consistently throughout the day.

Think Long-Term

Remember that you're not just changing how you eat today—you're investing in your health for decades to come. The nutritional choices you make in your 40s will influence how you feel in your 60s. The habits you establish in your 60s will determine your quality of life in your 80s.

Stay Flexible

Your nutritional needs will continue to evolve as you age. The approach that works for you now may need adjustments in five or ten years. Stay curious, keep learning, and be willing to adapt your approach as your body's needs change.

Seek Support

Don't try to do this alone. Work with healthcare providers who understand nutrition. Connect with family and friends who share your commitment to healthy aging. Join communities of people who are on similar journeys.

The Ripple Effect

When you start eating for your age, something interesting happens: the benefits extend far beyond your personal health. You become a role model for others. You show your children that aging doesn't have to mean decline. You demonstrate to your peers that it's never too late to make positive changes. You prove to yourself that you have more control over your health than you might have thought.

Margaret, the 87-year-old patient I mentioned in the introduction, often tells me that her commitment to eating for her age has inspired her entire family to make healthier choices. Her adult children have improved their diets, her grandchildren are more adventurous eaters, and her friends ask her for advice about healthy aging.

"I never thought I'd become the healthy eating guru of my social circle," she laughs. "But when people see that you can be energetic and healthy at 87, they want to know your secrets."

A Personal Message

As I finish writing this book, I'm reminded of why I became passionate about nutrition and aging in the first place. I've seen too many people accept decline as inevitable when it's actually optional. I've watched patients transform their health and vitality simply by understanding how to feed their bodies appropriately for their age.

But I've also learned that knowledge isn't enough. Information without action is just entertainment. The real magic happens when you take what you've learned and apply it consistently to your daily life.

You now have the knowledge. You understand how your nutritional needs change with age and what you should be eating at your current life stage. The question is: what will you do with this information?

I encourage you to start small, be consistent, and stay committed to the long-term view. Your future self is counting on the choices you make today.

The Promise of Ageless Vitality

Here's what I can promise you: if you apply the principles in this book consistently over time, you will age differently than you would have otherwise. You'll have more energy, better health, and a greater sense of control over your aging process.

You might not be able to stop time, but you can certainly slow its effects on your body and mind. You can be the person who surprises their doctor with their vitality. You can be the grandparent who keeps up with the grandchildren. You can be the

role model who shows others what's possible when you eat for
your age.

The choice is yours. The information is in your hands. The journey
to ageless vitality starts with your very next meal.

What will you choose?

Here's to your health, vitality, and successful aging.

Dr. Michael McCoy

www.ingramcontent.com/pod-product-compliance
Lightning Source LLC
Chambersburg PA
CBHW050038260726
48658CB00005B/1675